Distribution, publication, and copying in any form are prohibited and subject to damages.

TEN HYPNOSES

Copying, publishing, and sharing with third parties are only permitted with the written consent of the author. Please observe the notes on copyright and usage.

Distribution, publication, and copying in any form are prohibited and subject to damages.

Copying, publishing, and sharing with third parties are only permitted with the written consent of the author. Please observe the notes on copyright and usage.

Distribution, publication, and copying in any form are prohibited and subject to damages.

Ingo Michael Simon

TEN HYPNOSES

17

Exam Anxiety and Stage Fright

Copying, publishing, and sharing with third parties are only permitted with the written consent of the author. Please observe the notes on copyright and usage.

Distribution, publication, and copying in any form are prohibited and subject to damages.

© 2024 Ingo Michael Simon
All rights reserved.
Independently published
www.ingosimon.com

Important Notes for Urgent Attention:
The contents of this book are based on the practical experiences of the author with hypnosis applications and psychotherapy in a trance state. Although the author has strived for the utmost care, errors or misunderstandings in the presentation cannot be completely excluded. Therapeutic work with people and the application of hypnosis are solely the responsibility of the hypnotist. It cannot be ruled out that parts of this book may be misunderstood or that the application of a presented procedure may cause an undesirable reaction in the client. The author also assumes no co-responsibility if work with a client is carried out with reference to the statements in this book.

The Author:
Ingo Michael Simon studied psychology and education and is a hypnotherapist with practices in southwestern Germany and Switzerland. With the help of hypnosis-supported psychotherapy, he primarily treats people with persistent psychological conditions. His practice focuses on anxiety disorders, pathological compulsions, and psychosomatic illnesses. His therapeutic offerings mainly include classical and modern hypnosis applications and the dreamland therapy he developed himself.

Copying, publishing, and sharing with third parties are only permitted with the written consent of the author. Please observe the notes on copyright and usage.

Distribution, publication, and copying in any form are prohibited and subject to damages.

Notes on Copyright and Usage

Copying, publishing, and sharing with third parties is prohibited and only permitted with the written consent of the author. Please observe the following copyright and usage guidelines.

This work has been carefully crafted and created to the best of the author's knowledge and personal experience. It comprises text templates and application guidelines for professional hypnosis sessions. The author is a licensed psychotherapist with extensive experience in psychotherapy, coaching, and personal training using hypnotic techniques and methods. Nevertheless, the author and the publisher assume no liability for the accuracy of information, instructions, and advice, nor for any typographical errors. The author and publisher accept no responsibility or liability for the application of these texts and recommendations with clients or patients, nor for any potential consequences or unexpected reactions. It is expressly noted that the application of therapeutic and advisory techniques and formulations lies solely and entirely within the responsibility of the practitioner. This also applies to adherence to the boundaries of legally regulated medical and therapeutic practices. The fact that a book containing action proposals is freely available for sale does not imply that its application with clients or patients is permitted for everyone.

Copying, publishing, and sharing with third parties are only permitted with the written consent of the author. Please observe the notes on copyright and usage.

Distribution, publication, and copying in any form are prohibited and subject to damages.

Copying, publishing, and sharing with third parties are only permitted with the written consent of the author. Please observe the notes on copyright and usage.

Distribution, publication, and copying in any form are prohibited and subject to damages.

Table of Contents

Introduction 9
#1 11
#2 17
#3 22
#4 28
#5 34
#6 39
#7 44
#8 49
#9 54
#10 59
Overview of All Titles in the Series "Ten Hypnoses" 64

Copying, publishing, and sharing with third parties are only permitted with the written consent of the author. Please observe the notes on copyright and usage.

Distribution, publication, and copying in any form are prohibited and subject to damages.

Copying, publishing, and sharing with third parties are only permitted with the written consent of the author. Please observe the notes on copyright and usage.

Introduction

The series "Ten Hypnoses" is very well known in Germany, Austria, and Switzerland as a collection of texts for therapeutic work and is used by numerous psychotherapeutic practices, doctors, therapists, coaches, and other helping professionals. I am pleased to now be able to offer these texts in other countries as well.

Most therapists have their own methods for inducing and deepening trance as well as for exiting trance. Therefore, I have focused on the main part of the hypnosis. The texts in this book can be integrated as the main part into any hypnosis process.

The texts in this collection use various hypnosis techniques. I will not explain these in detail, as I assume that users have the appropriate training. It is also not necessary to understand the exact structure or functioning of the different parts. The texts can simply be read aloud, and they will have their effect.

Decide for yourself which text best suits your client or patient at any given time. You can also combine passages from different texts. It is not about using all ten hypnoses in sequence. It is a selection of possibilities.

I want to emphasize that books cannot replace therapy. Psychotherapy or other therapeutic treatments involve much more. A careful diagnosis is the necessary basis for deciding on the use of methods, including whether hypnosis or one of my texts should be used. Even in this case, preparatory discussions, follow-up discussions during the session, and of course, a therapeutic concept for the sequence of sessions and the content approaches are essential parts of therapy. This cannot and should not be achieved with a collection of texts.

In any case, I wish you much success in your work and I am pleased if my text templates can contribute in a small way.

Ingo Michael Simon

#1

Today, you are preparing to present yourself to others … … to show yourself and be the center of attention … … In the spotlight, you can feel secure and perform well because you are well-prepared … … Today, you will find all the skills and qualities you need for a successful presentation deep within yourself … … because deep inside you already have everything you need … … You know that all the important qualities and skills are already within you … … You know it and you are sure that everything you need for a successful presentation is already within you … … You can do it … … You already have all the skills you need to give a successful and confident presentation … … to present your expertise successfully … … to convince your audience … … to convince examiners … … to convince critics … … It's quite amazing how well you can adjust to presenting yourself successfully … … It comes naturally to you to present your topics and content in a way that excites your audience … … and it also comes naturally to you to show yourself in a way that impresses your audience … … It's truly remarkable how much potential each person has and how much we can find in a trance ... ... and it's amazing how much potential you already have and are discovering today ... ... Your body provides you with everything you need ... ... Strength and power are shown in the posture of your body ... ... Your inner self arranges everything for you and prepares you as if by itself for your presentation ... ... With each breath, your body adopts a more confident and stable posture ... ... the posture of a confident person, because that's what you can truly be ... ... a confident and good speaker ... ... who captivates and excites their audience ... ... You can do it, and your body shows you how ... ... You are relaxed and calm, and at the same time, your body takes on a commanding posture ... ... a posture that signals stability and assertiveness ... ... the posture of a winner ... ... Maybe you've already noticed that your body has changed ... ... that it has adopted a changed, stronger posture ... ...

... ... In your mind's eye, you look into a mirror ... ... You observe how your body straightens with each breath ... ... Your shoulders are straight ... ... your head slightly raised ... ... Your arms and legs have a constructive and proactive tension ... ... That's right ... ... You can imagine it very well ...

... watching yourself in the mirror and feeling this effect ... ... This is what winners look like ... ... And you are a winner ... ... confident and strong in your own conviction ... ... Exactly this conviction passes on to your audience ... ... Your gaze is firm ... ... your voice is stable, loud, and clearly audible ... ... And every eye contact from the audience shows you more clearly that you are full of self-confidence ... ... It's quite amazing how you manage to recognize every look from your audience as a confirmation of your quality ... ... Every question about your presentation confirms that your expertise is in demand and appreciated ... ... Every contribution from the audience proves that your presentation is interesting and invites them to learn more ... ... You spark interest in your audience ... ... It's really fun to listen to your presentation ... ... truly great how you stand there ... ... so impressive and confident ... ... so captivating and exciting is your presentation ... ... That's your success, that's how you imagined it and exactly how your presentation goes ... ... You present a topic ... ... and more than that ... ... You present yourself ... ... Really well done, how you do it ... ... and this success makes you stronger and stronger ... ... You see it clearly in front of you ... ... You are exceptionally good at it ... ... All your knowledge is available to you ... ... You draw from the depths of your knowledge and from the depths of your grown experience and competence ... ... Truly outstanding, how quickly your body adjusts to it ... ... how quickly your body has already adopted a changed, stronger posture ... ... This gives you the special gift of a confident appearance ... ... because deep inside you lies this confidence that you have been searching for ... ... deep inside you lies this strength that you have already found today ... ... You can use it every day ... ... whenever you want to present something or give a presentation, you find your own strength ... ... whenever you want to show something, you find your own strength ... ... whenever you want to convince, you find your own strength ... ... whenever you want to be successful, you find your own strength ... ... whenever you want to pass an exam, you find your own strength ... ... Your body provides you with everything you need for this ... ... Strength and power are shown in the posture of your body ... ... Your inner self arranges everything for you and prepares you as if by itself for your task/presentation/exam ... ... With each breath, your body adopts a more confident and stable posture ... ... the posture of a confident person, because that's what you can truly be … … a confident and good speaker … … who captivates and excites their audience … … You already can do it and your body shows you again and again how it works … … You are relaxed and calm and at the same time your body takes on a commanding posture … … a posture that signals stability and assertiveness … … the posture of a winner … … You are strong and confident … … You are very strong and very confident … … Today and every day … … The look in the inner mirror is a look into your own strength and power … … Today you have found your strength … … and what you achieve today, you can achieve on any other day of your life … … just like today … … exactly like today … …

Your deep inner self, your subconscious has already memorized this … … It has already saved the look into the inner mirror for you and understood … … A look into the inner mirror always shows you that you are truly strong, deep inside … … and that you can be just as strong on the outside … … Every look into a mirror reminds your subconscious immediately that you are strong deep inside and can be strong on the outside … … Even in the morning when you look into the mirror, your subconscious provides you with strength ... ... In any mirror you look at, it will be a look into the inner mirror, which is always a look into your strength ... ... into the strength that is already within you and helps you to present yourself and any topics you want to present convincingly ... ... Every look into a mirror reminds you that you are already strong ... ... so strong that you will indeed convince and be successful ... ...

#2

Today, you want to deal with your exam ... ... You want to pass it and more ... ... You want to feel good during the exam ... ... as good as possible ... ... as good as now ... ... You want to breathe calmly and recall your knowledge ... ... You want to speak fluently and feel calm hands ... ... as calm as now ... ... With each breath, you are now coming further to rest ... ... Each breath makes you calmer and more attuned to yourself ... ... Deep within you is this deep calm that you can feel now ... ... Deep within you, everything is in order ... ... Deep within you is all your knowledge ... ... Deep within you are all your abilities ... ... With each breath, you become aware of your own abilities ... ... You already have everything you need for a successful exam ... ... You can already do everything ... ... truly everything ... ... First, you realize how much you have already learned ... ... You have prepared long and intensively ... ... You have learned a lot and understood, you are really well prepared for your exam ... ... You calmly and serenely let what you have learned pass before your mind's eye once again ... ... Imagine your subject knowledge once again ... ... Think of the materials you used to prepare ... ... Perhaps you recall images ... ... mnemonics or important numbers ... ... Everything is well sorted ... ... So you can briefly recall and put away individual aspects or facts here and there ... ... can simply review what you have learned and be proud of having learned so much ... ... You can be really proud ... ... All your knowledge is ready to be recalled ... ... It is quite impressive how much you have learned and how well you have prepared yourself ... ... The more you focus on your slow, calm breathing, the more clearly you can feel the knowledge within you ... ... You can feel deep inside that there is a wealth of knowledge and competence ... ... like a vast ocean of knowledge within you ... ... You can fully trust that you are well prepared ... ... You have often passed exams ... ... You have repeatedly shown that you can succeed and achieve success ... ... You now let these successes flow into your consciousness ... ... You realize how successful you have already been and can always be again ... ... even with a calmer and better feeling ... ... You now recall images of successful exams ... ... perhaps some were not so bad in retrospect ... ... or they were difficult and exhausting, but your pride is all the greater because you really fought for success ... ... But again and again, you have succeeded ... ... again and again you have been successful ... ... you have fought through or fought back ... ... Focus on your breathing ... ... With each breath, you feel your own strength better ... ... With each breath, you feel the strength of all your small and big successes ... ... You feel the strength of easy successes and also of hard-won successes ... ... All successes were important ... ... All successes help you to be successful again ... ... You just let the images of your successes pass by ... ... and with the images of success come the feelings of success again ... ... Relief and pride ... ... Relief and pride ... ... You become even calmer inside ... ... Each breath lets you relax deeper ... ... You can now continue to prepare for your exam in all tranquility ... ... In calm and serenity, you now prepare for your exam ... ... It is easier than you thought before ... ... It is quite impressive how easily you can remember it ... ... In your imagination, you approach the exam day ... ... You take the good feeling you have in your relaxation now with you ... ... You anchor it deep inside you ... ... now and always ... ... You succeed now in staying calm and approaching the exam day ... ... You know that you have prepared well and that you have already had successes … … Then you approach the exam room … … With each breath, you come deeper to rest and a little closer to the room of the exam … … With each breath, you come to rest … … The closer you get to the exam room, the calmer you become today … … You come closer and closer and become calmer in the process … … It is quite impressive how calm you can be … … You focus entirely on the feeling of calm and serenity within you … … You stand in your thoughts in front of the exam room and are calm and serene … … Each breath makes you calmer … … Breathe calm into yourself before you enter the room … … Always when you exhale, you feel the calm particularly clearly … … always when you exhale … … So breathe out and enter the exam room … … Breathe out and enter the exam room … … With the feeling of calm and trust in your abilities, you enter the room … … You trust your abilities … … Orient yourself in the room and find your place … … With each step through the room, your confidence becomes stronger … … With each step through the room, you feel your own strength more … … You become stronger and find your place … … You settle in at your place with full confidence … … You breathe calmly and evenly and focus on your knowledge and abilities ... ... With each breath, your knowledge surfaces more and can be recalled by you ... ... You briefly close your eyes and take a deep breath in and slowly and long out ... ... and with exactly this breath, your subconscious immediately provides you with all your expertise ... ... With calm and serenity, you look forward to the exam ... ... You are strong and successful ... ... You feel it deep within you ... ... You are successful ... ...

Your subconscious saves this for you now ... ... As soon as you close your eyes to activate your expertise, you breathe deeply in and slowly and long out and immediately all your knowledge is available to you ... ... You can try it out while studying and make this connection stronger and stronger ... ... This way, you can check while studying that with one breath with closed eyes your expertise is actually activated and ready for you ... ... and in the exam, you do it exactly like this ... ... Close your eyes ... ... inhale and exhale and immediately all your expertise is available to you ... ...

#3

The following variant of a hypnosis main part works with an anchor in the form of sunglasses with blue lenses. An anchor is a trigger that is supposed to create a certain feeling or evoke a certain thought. We want to help the client to maintain a state free of anxiety in the exam with the help of sunglasses and to counteract the onset of exam anxiety. The best lenses are yellow, orange, or blue. Blue has proven to be the most effective in practice, as many students I prepared for exams with the help of the anti-anxiety glasses wore the glasses even during a written exam. Initially, the colored glasses were meant for preparation and to be taken off just before the actual exam. My clients found an even better way. In a state of relaxation, no fear can be felt, so we use a deep state of relaxation to set up the glasses as an anchor. We have the client open their eyes and look through the colored lenses while in a trance. Suggestively, we associate this color perception with the feeling of relaxation that is currently predominant. In everyday life, the client should then wear the glasses *repeatedly for a few hours during the learning phase; many have also decided to wear them continuously while reading and studying. The color perception is supposed to help prevent anxiety from arising. This approach may sound strange. Just try the colored glasses once. You might be surprised how well they are received and how well they usually work. The colored glasses can also be used for other fears, such as panic attacks (see Volume 14, Panic Attacks). By the way, you don't need special (and usually very expensive) color therapy glasses. Any sports glasses for joggers or cyclists are suitable. They are available for as little as 5 euros. Simply give your client the task of obtaining such glasses and bringing them along. They should wear them throughout the entire session.*

You have firmly resolved to reduce your exam anxiety … … You know the tension that arises and builds when the exam is approaching … … A fear that has often paralyzed you in exams … … You can train to control emerging fear, but you can do more … … You can ensure that it does not arise in the first place … … can ward it off before it even appears … … To do this, it is helpful to now reach a very deep state of relaxation … … You simply allow yourself to relax even more now … … sink even deeper … … sink deeper and deeper … … into a beautiful state of calm … … of deep inner calm … … and if you are tired, imagine you are starting to dream … … as if you were falling asleep … … just falling asleep … … to dream a beautiful dream … … in wonderful images that you can really enjoy … … beautiful images of calm and relaxation … … beautiful images of peace and quiet … … Everything becomes calm within you … … everything becomes very calm … … That's right … … just like that is good … … simply calm and relaxation … … deep calm and deep relaxation … … Now you feel good … … now nothing can burden or disturb you … … and if there should still be any disturbing thought, then you simply breathe it out … … It's as if you could simply breathe out any tension and any thought that might still be in the way and let it go … … with each breath, until you feel truly free and relaxed … … So breathe out for your inner calm … … Breathe out for your inner peace … … Breathe out for your relaxation … … Breathe out the fear … … Breathe out any thought of fear … … Breathe out any memory of fear … … Breathe out and come to rest … … Find deeper and deeper calm and relaxation … … deeper and deeper calm and relaxation ... ... So beautifully relaxed, everything is in order ... ... Your body can now learn to maintain this state of calm and free from fear permanently ... ... Your entire organism can learn this right now ... ... Focus on your feeling ... ... on this feeling of calm and relaxation that you are feeling right now ... ... The more you focus on the feeling of calm, the more clearly it becomes ... ... and now get ready to open your eyes and perceive the color of calm and serenity ... ... I will count to three, then you open your eyes ... ...

... ... [counting calmly, no pressure and no increased volume in the voice; it's not about leading out, but about fractionation.] ... ... one ... ... two ... ... three ... ... Open your eyes and perceive the color of calm and serenity ... ... Perceive this soothing blue (yellow/orange) very clearly and let this beautiful color flow deeply into your consciousness ... ... It becomes the color of your calming ... ... that's right ... ... very good ... ... Now close your eyes again and feel the soothing blue (yellow/orange) deeply within you ... ... that's right ... ... very good ... ...

Now feel the inner calm ... ... You can still feel it, perhaps even more clearly than before ... ... and at the same time, your deep inner self learns that this beautiful color is the color of your serenity ... ... the color of your inner calm ... ... This learning happens all by itself ... ... deep within you, it has already happened, your organism already knows that with the perception of the soothing color blue (yellow/orange) the feeling of calm is so important that you must feel it clearly ... ... So your own body immediately sends you this feeling of calm as soon as you perceive the color blue ... ... So let your body absorb this calming effect once more and make it real ... ... I will count to three again for you, then you can open your eyes again and absorb even more of the beautiful color of your calming ... ... [counting calmly, no pressure and no increased volume in the voice; it's not about leading out, but about fractionation.] ... ... one ... ... two ... ... three ... ... Open your eyes and perceive the color of your calming ... ... Perceive this soothing blue (yellow/orange) very clearly and let this relaxing color flow deeply into your consciousness ... ... It becomes the color of your calm ... ... that's right ... ... very good ... ... Now close your eyes again and feel the calming blue (yellow/orange) deeply within you ... ... that's right ... ... very good ... ...

Your body now knows that there is your calm color, which is also your anti-fear color … … and whenever you wear the glasses through which you are now looking, and then perceive this soothing color, your organism immediately remembers the important calm you need … … and whenever you look through the glasses, your deep inner self immediately provides you with the feeling of calm as best and as strongly as it can … … With all its might, calm arises in you when you look through the glasses you are wearing now … … Every day calm … … every day … … just like now … … exactly like now … …

#4

The following hypnosis session works with an olfactory anchor (scent anchor). An anchor is a trigger that is supposed to create a certain feeling or evoke a certain thought. We want to help the client to enter a calm state with the help of a specific scent. The approach is very suitable for exam anxiety as well as stage fright for actors or speakers. We discuss the procedure with the client before the session and keep a vial with a scent ready. This can be a smelling oil or an aroma spray that the client should only smell in a trance. During the hypnosis session, we set up the anchor by presenting the scent and associating it suggestively. The scent itself should not be too strong but does not have to be particularly pleasant for the client. It depends on the suggestive association. However, it should not be experienced as repulsive either. With mild aroma oils, this is rarely the case.

Staying calm and composed is your goal ... ... You have firmly resolved to see exams/performances/presentations as challenges and to face these challenges … … always finding the strength within yourself to control the fear … … overcoming your fear again and again and moving forward … … confronting your tasks with pride and a sense of security … … You have succeeded time and time again … … because you did not give up, you fought back after setbacks … … But today you can work on handling it more easily … … Today you can do something about the fear … … Today you can work on your success … …

… … We are working with an anchor today, we've already discussed it … … Perhaps you are already wondering how quickly this anchor will work … … how fast it will be for the scent you are about to experience to calm you and give you a good feeling of strength … … It may surprise you how well this anchor works … … how quickly you can actually enter a calm feeling just before the exam/performance, even and especially when it gets difficult … …

… … Today is the first day of your new life … … a life in which you succeed in quickly entering a calm state … … The good thing is that it is much easier than you thought before … … Perhaps you wonder how best and quickest you can immediately feel calm and inner strength … … feel courage and the will to succeed ... ... It is easier than you thought ... ... To do this, you now go mentally to a time when you felt really good, perhaps to the best time of your life ... ... perhaps it was a long period, a few years ... ... or it was a short time that was really beautiful ... ... a vacation, an experience ... ... maybe just a very short moment, but one that was really beautiful ... ... the best moment of your life ... ... if you want, just take the best fantasy of your life ... ... and go completely into this feeling associated with it ... ... feel once again how beautiful it was ... ... The more you focus on your memory or your fantasy, the more intensely you can feel the good feeling ... ... Then you also recall a success ... ... perhaps an exam you passed or a performance with a lot of applause ... ... That felt good ... ... You did it and feel proud ... ... joy ... ... happiness ... ... You feel really good in this memory ... ... or in this fantasy ... ... You feel better and better ... ... The more you focus on your memory or your fantasy, the more intensely you can feel the good feeling that comes with success ... ... just like that ... ... Let the feeling become more beautiful within you ... ... Exactly this feeling is what you need ... ... Exactly this feeling you need every day ... ... You can secure it ... ... You can make sure it works in your waking life as well … … just like now … … every day just like now … … It's very simple … … You can go into this feeling every day and feel good then … … You succeed again and again, even and especially when it gets difficult … … also just before the exam/performance … … Then it suddenly becomes easy to feel the good feeling … … Then it suddenly becomes easy to manage your task/s and be successful … … [Open the vial with the aroma and move it towards the client's nose; hold it there] … …

… … Now take a deep breath and consciously perceive the scent you are smelling … … a pleasant scent … … at the same time you feel very clearly that you are indeed calm … … and if you now pay close attention to your feeling, you will also notice that you become even calmer with this scent … … Your good feeling and the scent you perceive now combine … … They belong together … … This scent and calm belong very closely together … … This scent means: Yes, I stay calm and I am successful! … … Yes, I stay calm and I am successful! … … Take another deep breath … … The scent of success spreads within you … … The scent of success flows through your entire body … … from the nose to the lungs … … into the upper body … … into the belly and legs ... ... Calm and courage flow through you completely ... ... Calm and courage flow through you completely ... ...

... ... And whenever you smell this scent, you feel calm immediately ... ... Whenever you perceive exactly this scent, you feel very clearly that you are becoming calmer ... ... Even when you only think of the scent, you can already feel that you are becoming calmer ... ... Your subconscious imprints this scent and associates it with the beautiful feeling of calm and success ... ... Calm and success ... ... [Now remove and close the vial] ... ...

... ... Keep breathing calmly and enjoy the calm ... ... Give yourself now mindfulness and attention and trust your subconscious to support you, always getting into this calm state quickly again by simply smelling the vial with the scent I just presented to you ... ...

You can even test it ... ... As soon as you perceive the scent, you feel good and become calm ... ... It's as if you are breathing in calm and success when you smell it ... ... Smelling this scent means breathing in calm and success ... ...

… … [Open the vial again and hold it near the client's nose so they can clearly perceive the scent; hold briefly and then close again] … …

… … That feels good … … very, very good … … Your inner self imprints very firmly that already the grip on the vial with your personal success scent triggers the signal in your body: Yes, I stay calm and I am successful! … … Yes, I stay calm and I am successful! … …

#5

You know the fear before and during exams … … the fear of failure, the fear of being judged poorly … … the fear of embarrassing yourself … … Today you want to do something about it, you want to free yourself from the fear … … Perhaps you wonder how quickly it might be possible to let go of such a fear … … Perhaps you have already imagined how nice it would be if you could do it like others who simply go into exams without fear … … Possibly the fearless ones are a bit nervous, tense … … That's good because without tension the memory isn't as good either … … But you know people who don't know exam fear … … They just go into the exam and do it … … go through with it and then pass … … If you think about others, you probably come up with some who pass exams more easily … … You think of some who have no exam fear … … You think of some who master the exams coldly or confidently … … You know as much as they do … … You can do as much as they can … … Maybe you can even do more … … If you manage to recall your knowledge in the exam like they do, you will also pass your exams and feel better ... ... If you manage to present your skills and abilities in the exam because you are calmer, you will also pass your exam and feel better ... ... Surely you even know a person who can do it exceptionally well ... ... someone who always passes ... ... someone who has no fear ... ... Possibly this person even finds exams quite good because he or she can present their own expertise there ... ... You know such a person ... ... among those who master exams confidently, there is one person who could be a role model for you ... ... a person you would say, "I should be able to do it like that too!" ... ... Maybe a sympathetic person, someone you like very much ... ... Sometimes it's different though ... ... Sometimes it's someone we don't like very much, but who can be a role model ... ... a role model just for exams, that's enough ... ... You find such a person in your memory and can learn from them today ... ... Perhaps you wonder how it is possible to simply learn from someone to be calmer and more determined ... ... to remain confident with a constructive tension ... ... Focus on your body feeling and feel the calm and relaxation now ... ... Maybe you want to relax even deeper ... ... let go even more and become calmer ... ... completely calm ... ... Then you imagine this exam role model ... ... Let their image appear before your mind's eye ... ... Imagine how this person looks ... ... Then imagine meeting this person just before an exam that only they have to take ... ... You are completely calm and relaxed ... ... Your role model too because this person has exams under control ... ... Imagine you can go into the exam room with this role model and watch them pass the exam... ... Let the image appear before your mind's eye ... ... Look closely ... ... Pay attention to the posture ... ... See how your role model stands there ... ... and also pay attention to the movements ... ... Every movement shows strength and expressiveness ... ... Observe your role model's body and feel the same strength, the same possibility of movement in your own body ... ... You can do it too ... ... You watch it today and practice it ... ... Then pay attention to the facial expression ... ... Look at the facial expressions ... ... and feel the same movements in your own face ... ... Feel how good it feels to be so confident and calm in the exam ... ... Your role model can do it ... ... You can do it ... ... You can do it ... ... You learn from your role model today how it works ... ... You just have to watch and everything happens by itself ... ... Continue to look at your role model ... ... but you can do more ... ... You can see through your role model's eyes ... ... slip into this

person like a spirit and see through their eyes ... ... So watch how your role model experiences the exam, completely different from you before ... ... Your role model sees examiners who pose no threat ... ... Your role model sees the examiners as allies on the path of learning and passing ... ... That's how you see it too, because you are looking through the role model's eyes now and see everything exactly the same ... ... and feel the same confidence and strength ... ... Now you also feel the body feeling of the role model better because you stand in their shoes ... ... in their place ... ... That's how it feels ... ... Your role model can do it ... ... You can do it ... ... You can do it exactly the same way ... ... here and today in your imagination, it is very easy ... ... and later in your waking life, it is just as easy because you already know how it works ... ... You have already learned it ... ... Your role model can do it ... ... You can do it too ... ... So you learn more and more to go into the exam just like your role model ... ... So you learn more and more to be just as strong and calm as your role model ... ... So you learn more and more to be just as confident and sovereign as your role model ... ... So you go more and more into this good and strong feeling that you are feeling now ... ... You make your role model's behavior your own ... ... You just do it exactly like this person, whoever it may be ... ... You pass exams just like this person ... ... exactly like that ... ... You have already learned it ... ... You can already do it ... ...

This learning process takes place deep inside you ... ... deep in your feeling ... ... and exactly there every pattern of your role model's movements and exam behavior is laid out as your own pattern ... ... So you can access it exactly when you want to ... ... Your deep inner self continues to learn for you ... ... Your subconscious continues to learn, exactly how to be successful in exams like your role model ... ... Whenever you meet this person or think of them, it is a signal for your subconscious to learn as much exam strength as possible from this role model ... ... So you take on more and more clearly the confidence and sovereignty of your role model in exam situations ... ... This makes you successful in your exams ... ...

Distribution, publication, and copying in any form are prohibited and subject to damages.

Copying, publishing, and sharing with third parties are only permitted with the written consent of the author. Please observe the notes on copyright and usage.

#6

Today you are preparing for your presentation ... ... You know that good preparation is particularly important ... ... because well-prepared it is easy for you to present your presentation calmly and with an overview ... ... You then feel confident and good ... ... more than that, it can even be really fun to give your talk ... ... You have long prepared yourself for your presentation and the presentation tools ... ... But today it is about inner preparation because that is especially important ... ... Today's preparation helps you to actually retrieve what you have to offer ... ... to retrieve what you have in terms of expertise ... ... to retrieve what you have in terms of experience ... ... to retrieve what you have in terms of personality and charisma ... ... and that is more than you thought ... ... To do this, you pack your presentation case ... ... your very own presentation and presentation case ... ... It lies before you, a sturdy case that protects its contents well so that you can access them unscathed at any time when you need something from this case ... ... Choose the sturdiest case you can imagine ... ...

perhaps made of sturdy plastic … … or of aluminum … … choose it the way it seems most stable to you … … Imagine your presentation case as intensely as possible … … until you have a clear image of how your presentation case should look … … Very good … …

… … Now open the case … … It is completely empty … … You can determine what should be in this case … … because in this special case you can pack your own feelings and abilities to access them exactly when you need them most … … to access them exactly when you give a talk … … when you present yourself and your offer … … You start by filling the case … … with your own abilities, with your potential … … with all your experience … … with your know-how … … perhaps with your tips and tricks for a successful presentation or a contract or completion that will result from it … … To do this, pack five special items into your case … … Five items that represent five skills and qualities for you … … Choose an item or a symbol for your expertise … … Knowledge is power … … Knowledge creates an advantage … … Your knowledge is an important key to success … … Truly remarkable how much expertise you actually have … … Decide now on an item that represents this expertise … …

[Wait ten seconds, then continue reading] ... ... Put this item in the case ... ... Put your knowledge and expertise in the case ... ... As soon as you close and take the case with you, your expertise is fully and quickly available to you at any time ... ... [Wait ten seconds, then continue reading] ... ... Now choose an item or a symbol for your experience ... ... You have often experienced situations where you had to prove something ... ... Situations where you had to present something and present yourself ... ... in exams ... ... in presentations ... ... or in discussions ... ... Experience gives confidence ... ... Experience means flexibility ... ... Your experience is an important key to success ... ... Truly remarkable how much experience you actually have ... ... Decide now on an item that represents this experience ... ... [Wait ten seconds, then continue reading] ... ... Put this item in the case ... ... Put your entire experience in your case ... ... As soon as you close and take the case with you, your experience is fully and quickly available to you at any time ... ... [Wait ten seconds, then continue reading] ... ... Next, choose an item or a symbol for your charisma ... ... Charisma is the aura of the winner ... ... Charisma captivates listeners ... ... Your charisma is an important key to success ... ...

Perhaps you have already thought about how it was also your charisma that contributed to your successes ... ... to all the big and also the small successes ... ... Perhaps you also thought it was always just knowledge and skills that advanced you ... ... But when you think about it closely, you also recognize that it is often the charisma that makes us successful ... ... the effect outward ... ... the charisma ... ... Truly remarkable how much charisma you actually have ... ... Decide now on an item that represents this charisma ... ... [Wait ten seconds, then continue reading] ... ... Put this item in the case ... ... Put your charisma in the case ... ... As soon as you close and take the case with you, your charisma is fully and quickly available to you at any time ... ... [Wait ten seconds, then continue reading] ... ... Now choose an item or a symbol for your oratory skills ... ... Oratory is the special talent that counts ... ... Oratory captivates listeners and convinces them ... ... Your oratory is an important key to success ... ... Truly remarkable how much oratory you actually have ... ... Decide now on an item that represents this oratory ... ... [Wait ten seconds, then continue reading] ... ... Put this item in the case ... ... Put your oratory in the case ... ... [Wait ten seconds, then continue reading] ... ... As soon as you close and take the case with you, your oratory is fully and quickly available to you at any time … … [Wait ten seconds, then continue reading] … … Now choose an item or a symbol for success … … Success is your goal … … Success is your goal … … Quite remarkable how often you have been successful, how much potential for success you have … … Decide now on an item that represents success … … [Wait ten seconds, then continue reading] … … Put this item in the case … … As soon as you close and take the case with you, your success is assured … …

You always have your case with you … … As soon as you start your presentation, your case opens by itself and provides you with all the good qualities immediately and fully … … Expertise … … Experience … … Charisma … … Oratory … … and Success … …

#7

Ideomotoric refers to the phenomenon that our body follows our feelings and thoughts with movements. In everyday life, this following is shown as posture, muscle tension, and movement patterns of a person, which naturally change with the mood and thoughts. In trance, ideomotoric signals can be used to obtain information that the client cannot actively communicate. For example, the subconscious can answer questions with an agreed finger signal. Of course, ideomotoric reactions can also be used suggestively, for example, with arm levitations and catalepsy. Such an approach, which I also use in the following text, strengthens trust in hypnosis and in one's own ability to change and thus promotes therapy.

Today you want to let go of your exam fear/stage fright ... ... You have dealt with how all this could have happened, how this fear actually arose ... ... Perhaps you have found some good answers to it ... ... possibly also realizing that long-past fears of failure are still within you today ... ... and have shown themselves in exam situations or in performances or presentations ... ... But no matter how the fear arose, it is about how you can let it go ... ... This is possible even without knowing exactly how it could arise ... ... Fear is like a pattern ... ... like a learned routine ... ... It is there, even though it actually belongs to an earlier time, namely the time when it arose, whenever that was ... ... Back then, it had a function, then it became independent and stayed ... ... Now it is time to change that ... ... Your body can help you with this ... ... Our body can give us important signals and clues, can show us what is going on deep in our emotions ... ... Your body can also show you that you are letting go of an old thought pattern ... ... You have already succeeded in your thoughts, and that is really good ... ... Now you can work on letting go of your fear feelings ... ... Your deep inner self does this for you ... ... Your subconscious can plan anew for you and thus ensure that you remain calmer from the start and that fear does not arise in the first place ... ... To do this, you must allow your subconscious to help you ... ... and that is exactly what you have already done by focusing on your inner calm and your body ... ... So you have already sent your subconscious the message that it may now work for you in peace … … a beautiful idea that it is not you who works once, but your unconscious side … … quietly … … You allow it and that is why it is possible … Now focus your attention on your hands … … Check once again that they are lying properly beside your body … … loose and comfortable … … in complete relaxation … … Your palms are lightly touching the surface … …

… [If this position has not been taken or has changed in the meantime, please correct it until the hands are lying loosely beside the body.] …

Now your subconscious takes the lead … … Your deep inner self ensures that old thought and behavior patterns that produced your exam fear/stage fright fall away from you and that new thoughts of calm and confidence are built up … … without any effort … … in peace and quiet … … Your subconscious ensures that you treat yourself and your inner resources more mindfully and lets this new mindfulness and care become a matter of course … … It is like an inner cleansing … … Old patterns of thinking and acting are let go … … new patterns of thinking and acting are built up and help you to remain calm from now on and to control nervousness … … to let go of emerging fear early and sustainably … … to work with calm and overview … … to shape your exams/performances with confidence in inner guidance … …

… … Your subconscious now shows you how quickly it progresses in this cleansing and creation … … You will recognize it by the fact that your hands begin to turn outwards … … Your hands slowly turn outwards until they finally lie on their backs … … Focus on your hands and just let it happen … … Your subconscious now begins to turn your hands outwards … … slowly, at your speed, at your pace … … The more you internally adjust to your new thinking and behavior, the more your hands turn … … The more you adjust to truly letting go of your fear, the more your hands turn … … They turn more and more outwards … … Your hands turn with each step of internal change and realignment … … just like that … … Feel how your hands slowly turn … … They turn outwards … … as if by themselves … … You don't have to do anything … … You don't have to do anything actively … … You don't have to change anything actively … … Your subconscious does everything necessary for you … … And as a sign of letting go of your fear thoughts, your hands turn … … more and more … … more and more … … until they show with the palms upwards … …

… [Observe the turning of the hands, which sets in relatively quickly. The client connects the turning with inner change. Repeat suggestions about the turning of the hands until they lie on their backs on the surface.] …

Isn't it amazing how quickly your subconscious is willing to help you and even show it to you … Your inner self tells you: Yes, I am reorienting myself … Yes, I am letting go of the old fear feelings now … Yes, I give myself mindfulness and care … Yes, I take good care of myself from now on … Yes, I am and remain calm … Yes, I am and remain calm …

… … Your inner self firmly imprints that you are now free and can go new ways … … and whenever you want to strengthen the feeling of inner calm, you can simply lay your hands beside your body and consciously turn them … … In doing so, you breathe out deeply and then feel the inner liberation, the letting go of all fear feelings … … You can do this any day of your life if you want … … whenever you

**want ... ... and wherever you want ... ... It is very simple ...
...**

#8

Today you are here to deal with your old thought patterns and everything that led to your stage fright/exam fear ... ... Everything that lies deep in our feelings can also be felt in our bodies ... ... Every thought, every mood ... ... every single feeling manifests in our bodies ... ... shows itself there as a feeling of pressure ... ... as tension ... ... as an indescribable feeling ... ... sometimes even as a queasy feeling or pain ... ... or just as a strange tingling ... ... So if you can feel your body clearly, you can achieve everything you have set out to do ... ... understand everything ... ... and change everything ... ...

... ... Somewhere in your body lies the old thought patterns that led to your stage fright/exam fear ... ... Let's call it best your fear pattern ... ... It sits deep within you and acts from there without you noticing it ... ... But by now you know it ... ... You have long recognized that there is this special pattern ... ... You have accepted that it is there ... ... At the same time, you have set out to find it and then dissolve it ... ...

...... It is anchored in your feelings and thoughts but also in your body ...... You can feel it in your body ...... Maybe you know that you can feel everything that belongs to you physically if you come to rest, as you do now ...... and focus on your body ...... as you do now ...... Your body stores everything for you ...... every event and every feeling imprints itself in your body like a memory ...... Of course, you have experienced in your everyday life how your fear pattern can have an effect, but it also shows itself in your body ...... just differently ...... as tension ...... as warmth or cold ...... as pressure or in another way ...... All thought patterns that we carry deep within us show up at a specific point in our body most clearly ...... as a signal that we can perceive ...... So your fear pattern also shows up in your body as a signal that can warn you ...... so you don't fall into the trap of overwhelming fear again ...... so you can take better care of yourself and react in time ...... You just have to recognize this spot, then you can work on it and build a new pattern ......

...... Now focus your attention on your body and feel your body ...... Scan from head to toe as if with a scanner and find this special spot ...... Find this spot that feels different somehow because your fear pattern sits there … … You find it … … It feels different … … maybe just a bit colder or warmer … … maybe as a tingling … … or as a slight goosebump that suddenly forms … … Wherever this spot is … … There your fear pattern shows itself through a physical signal … … right there … … But even if you didn't find it … … It's there … … Then just take the spot that comes to your mind spontaneously … … wherever that is … …

… … Feel deeper and deeper there … … Go entirely into this feeling … … however it may be … … It is your fear/stage fright that you feel there … … Go deeper and deeper into this spot of your body and feel the signals of your body more clearly … … Maybe it feels exhausting or burdensome … … Maybe you thought you had already overcome it more … … Don't worry, because here you feel above all the thought pattern that led to your exam fear/stage fright … …

… … Now focus all your attention and all your mindfulness and loving care on exactly this point of your body and connect with the inner pattern that lies there … … Imagine how from this spot a warm feeling flows in all directions … … as if there were a small healing spring at exactly this spot, which spreads its healing water and warmth gently in all directions ... ... Let it become more and more pleasant, as pleasant as possible ... ... Imagine healing water or better yet a beautiful balm that flows from the spring and spreads throughout your body ... ... Let this spot of your body become a healing spring and work more and more pleasantly for you ... ... The healing warmth of the balm can encompass your entire body because you bring this mindfulness ... ... this turning towards yourself ... ... So this spot of your body becomes calmer ... ... more and more relaxed ... ... more and more pleasant ... ... and just as pleasantly the thought pattern changes ... ... More and more old entanglements dissolve and are replaced by new thought patterns of self-love and mindfulness ... ... Everywhere where the fear pattern was recently, you find more and more love from you for yourself ... ... more and more love from you for yourself ... ... your self-love and mindfulness ... ... your self-love and mindfulness ... ... Breathe calmly and evenly and trust in the power within you ... ... Everywhere where the fear pattern was recently, you find more and more love from you for yourself ... ... more and more love from you for yourself ... ... your self-love and mindfulness ... ... your self-love and mindfulness ... ...

... ... You feel the change in your body and realize that your body can always show you how you are feeling emotionally ... ... especially the feelings that you couldn't always feel so well in everyday life ... ... Now you can, because you know that your body helps you ... ... So you pay attention to your body every day and already ask yourself in the morning when you get up how your body feels today ... ... It shows you what you need to pay attention to ... ... Whenever you find a spot that feels significantly different from the rest of your body, you give yourself mindfulness and focus on this spot ... ... In doing so, you connect with the feeling that lies within you and recognize it ... ... This way, you can react ... ... This way, you can recognize in time when you need to take better care of yourself ... ... This way, fear doesn't arise at all ... ... This way, your stage fright/exam fear dissolves ... ...

#9

Today we are taking a journey together ... ... a journey that is only possible because you can dive deep into your imagination ... ... because you have access to your creativity and find the way inward ... ... In your dreams, you can think of everything that is possible or seemingly impossible ... ... But usually, much more is possible than we think because imagination and reality are very close together, so close that we sometimes can't really separate them ... ... and don't have to separate them because every daydream can also become truth when the right time comes ... ... Maybe the right time is today ... ... right now, at this very moment ... ... So you direct your attention and mindfulness to the center of your body, where your gut feeling is, and imagine that you could sink with your entire perception into this point ... ... sinking deeper and deeper into yourself to be completely in your feeling ... ... to arrive in the land of your dreams now ... ... You stand in front of a cinema and look at the sign above the entrance that says "Cinema of Life" ... ... The door opens by itself, and you go inside ... ... You enter a large cinema hall that is completely empty ... ... No one but you is here ... ... You can choose a seat ... ... You find a nice comfortable seat in a plush cinema chair ... ... You find a seat in the cinema of life that gives you a very good view ... ... a seat from which you can see the screen best ... ... in the best distance or the best closeness you need ... ... You make yourself comfortable, and you think about how it could have happened that such great fear and insecurity arose ... ... When you feel the fear today, you don't really know why it's there ... ... why it comes up in certain situations ... ... when you are in the spotlight ... ... when you want or have to prove something ... ... when you are seen ... ... when you are judged ... ... And while you are still thinking about it, it slowly gets darker in the cinema of life ... ... The light slowly goes out because the show is about to begin ... ... a performance just for you ... ... Slowly the curtain in front of the screen opens ... ... It slowly reveals the screen and with it the view into your deep feeling ... ... into the feeling of back then, a time long past, when you were also judged ... ... Back then, you had no chance ... ... back then, the judgment was already made before you could really do anything ... ... The screen lights up ... ... and slowly images from a time long ago, a long-past and sometimes forgotten time, appear ... ... Images that show you how it was back then ... ... as a child ... ... when you were in the spotlight because you were judged ... ... maybe it was more like being condemned ... ... You were afraid back then ... ... Just watch, the images show themselves on their own ... ... maybe images of an embarrassing situation ... ... maybe at school or at home ... ... and possibly they are also images of your past everyday life ... ... Images that show you that you were under pressure back then ... ... Maybe you experienced violence, or you could never please one or more people ... ... experienced repeatedly not being enough ... ... But that was not your own thought ... ... You wanted to be accepted and loved ... ... But the recognition and affection you sought you didn't find in that way ... ... You needed someone to tell you that you are lovable and good, even if you don't deliver a special performance once ... ... even if something goes wrong once ... ... But back then, it turned out differently ... ... You experienced judgments that slowly became your own because you heard or felt them so often ... ... Then you started to believe yourself that you were not good enough ... ... that you would fail or were a failure ... ... Your fear could arise like this ... ... The images on the screen in the cinema of your life show you how it was back then ... ... They also show you the people who contributed to it because you lived with them ... ... Some you know well, others may not even have a face on the screen up front because there are also people who made a contribution to your life without you really noticing ... ... You look at everything in peace, immerse yourself in the past ... ... and you realize that the past cannot be changed ... ... even if some people intentionally treated you badly or wanted to keep you down ... ... It happened as it did ... ... It is part of your life story ... ... You don't have another one ... ... You watch the images today to learn anew inside because today you learn from the same situations and people how to keep calm when you are in the spotlight ... ... Today you learn from your own past and your own life story to let go of exam fear/stage fright because your fear belongs to a time long past ... ... today you can be calm and strong ... ... You have already learned it ... ... Maybe the images you see fill you with anger ... ... or with disappointment and sadness ... ... Watch them and prepare to let them go, to give everything that once happened to the past and to detach yourself from it ... ... it's over ... ... You don't have to forgive anyone … … it's enough if you can let go … … And you do that in the land of dreams by closing the curtain on the screen … … You decide it like that and at the same moment the curtain draws in front of the images … … They remain in the film of your life because you can't erase your past … … But with the curtain you are now closing, you are making the deep inner decision to leave the fear that belongs to the past there … … and your exam fear/stage fright belongs to the past … …

Then you lean back in your cinema chair … … In your mind's eye, you see yourself free from exam fear/stage fright and inwardly light … … In your imagination, you have already let go of the fear, have given it to the past in the cinema of your life, where it belongs … … but imagination and reality are very close together, and in the land of dreams, both are the same … … So you can also let go of the fear in your waking life … … You have already let it go there too … … Then you think about the fact that the land of dreams is deep inside you … … It has always been there … … I'm just telling you about it …

#10

In our imagination, we can do anything … … There are no limits that can hold us back, only the limit of our own belief and our own creativity … … But even in waking life, it is the limits of our beliefs, our convictions, that hold us back or restrict us … … We can all do much more than we think … … You can do much more than you think … … So I invite you to a journey in your imagination … … Only what you can think can also happen … … Only what is possible in your imagination can actually become true … … and deep in your imagination, in your dreams, you can already let go of the fear today … … Just focus on your breathing and feel how your breath flows in and out … … While doing so, you can already imagine leaving your body, gliding away like the wind of your breath, and fully entering your imagination … … into the land of your dreams … … a land of unlimited possibilities and visions … … You have already dealt with your fears and know the fear before and in situations where you are on the spot … … perhaps in exams or in presentation situations … … in performances and presentations ... ... If you think about it now, you realize that it has always been like that when you were in the spotlight and the eyes and criticism were directed at you ... ... That was often the case, but now it is already different ... ... You have already taken important steps ... ... decided to face the fear ... ... finally get out of it and confidently pass your exams/presentations/performances ... ... To do this, you have considered the fear, found out what it does to you, and started to let it go ... ... Today, you can take a significant step and finally let go of the rest of your fear of exams/presentations/performances ... ... I am taking you on a journey ... ... a journey into and through your imagination ... ... Perhaps you know that your imagination always shows you only what you can actually do ... ... and you can let go of your exam fear or stage fright completely today ... ... You can let go of the fear ... ... You want to let go of the fear ... ... and you will let go of the fear ... ... here and today ... ... Imagine you are standing on a high mountain ... ... It is the mountain of demands and challenges ... ... You are here at the top for a very special reason ... ... You want to let go of your exam fear, your stage fright ... ... to be precise, only the rest of this fear, because you have already overcome a lot, as you have started to deal with your fear ... ...

You breathe in deeply and out and feel how your chest expands with each breath ... ... The feeling of freedom becomes stronger within you ... ... Then you put both hands together as if in prayer ... ... And every thought of fear flows from your head to your shoulders, further to your arms, and finally into your hands ... ... All memories of fear flow to your hands ... ... Every idea of fear flows to your hands ... ... Every notion that fear, which has already disappeared, could come back flows to your hands ... ... Every fear of being in the spotlight flows to your hands ... ... Exam fear ... ... Fear during presentations ... ... Stage fright during performances or presentations ... ... Every fear flows to your hands ... ... Now ... ... Every single thought of fear flows to your hands ... ... Now ... ... If you focus on your body feeling and perceive your body with much mindfulness and fully consciously, you can even feel the flow of the fear thoughts ... ... from the head to the shoulders ... ... to the arms and down to the hands ... ... Between your hands, a sphere of your fear thoughts forms ... ... Every remaining bit of fear that might still be in you flows to your hands and forms a sphere there

… … firm and smooth the sphere feels, like a glass sphere … … the sphere of your fears … … This sphere gets bigger and firmer because all thoughts of fear flow into it … … Every memory of fear flows into the sphere between your hands … … Every notion that fear could arise again flows into this sphere between your hands … … Finally, all thoughts of fear arrive in the sphere and you feel completely free … … Here in the land of dreams, everything is possible … … Here you can separate the fear from yourself and let it go as a sphere … … But everything that is possible here in the land of dreams is also possible in your waking life … … Also in your waking everyday life, you can let go of the fear … … just like here … … Look at the sphere … … a firm and stable sphere of fear … … It is outside your body and no longer belongs to you … … And now you take the sphere and throw it in a high arc down the slope to finally let go of your fear … … You let it go and it rolls down the mountain … … rolls further and further away from you, moving away inexorably … … Your fear disappears faster and faster … … and with it also every notion of returning fear … … Every thought of fear rolls down into the valley … … It rolls into the valley, so far away that you can no longer see it … … You have completely freed yourself from your fear … … here and today … … once and for all … … You have freed yourself from exam fear … … here and today … … once and for all … … once and for all … … You feel free and secure … … calm and courageous … … strong and independent … … ready for every challenge … … confident in every exam … … confident in every presentation … … confident in every talk … … confident in every performance … …

You feel the sense of freedom and relief deep within you … … and your mood slowly becomes happier and more relaxed … … Here in the land of dreams, everything is possible, even the release from fear … … also the rediscovery of your own strength and self-confidence, which now take the place that was previously occupied by fear … … Self-confidence replaces fear … … now … … Self-confidence replaces fear … … now … … Then you think about the fact that the land of dreams is deep inside you … … It has always been there … … I'm just telling you about it …

Distribution, publication, and copying in any form are prohibited and subject to damages.

Overview of All Titles in the Series "Ten Hypnoses"

Volume 1: Smoking Cessation
Volume 2: Anxiety and Restlessness
Volume 3: Burnout
Volume 4: Reducing Overweight
Volume 5: Coping with the Past
Volume 6: Suicidal Thoughts and Attempts
Volume 7: Psycho-Oncology
Volume 8: Obsessions and Tics
Volume 9: Self-Confidence and Decision-Making
Volume 10: Grief Work
Volume 11: Psychosomatics
Volume 12: Chronic Pain
Volume 13: Depressive Thoughts
Volume 14: Panic Attacks
Volume 15: Domestic Violence, Victim Support
Volume 16: Post-Traumatic Stress
Volume 17: Exam Anxiety and Stage Fright
Volume 18: Anti-Violence Training, Offender Support
Volume 19: Addiction Tendencies
Volume 20: Social Phobia and Fear of Contact
Volume 21: Nail Biting
Volume 22: Self-Awareness and Self-Love
Volume 23: Teeth Grinding and Night Clenching
Volume 24: Feelings of Guilt
Volume 25: Fear in Crowds
Volume 26: Fear of Flying, Aviophobia
Volume 27: Fear in Enclosed Spaces, Claustrophobia
Volume 28: Tinnitus, Ear Noises
Volume 29: Fear of Heights
Volume 30: Neurodermatitis

Copying, publishing, and sharing with third parties are only permitted with the written consent of the author. Please observe the notes on copyright and usage.

Volume 31: Finding Inner Balance
Volume 32: Overcoming Loneliness
Volume 33: Fear of Illness, Hypochondria
Volume 34: Anticipatory Anxiety, Fear of Fear
Volume 35: Jealousy in Relationships
Volume 36: Driving Anxiety
Volume 37: New Start after Separation
Volume 38: Fear of Injections
Volume 39: Heart Anxiety Neurosis
Volume 40: Overcoming Resentment and Anger
Volume 41: Resolving Blockages and Positive Thinking
Volume 42: Stress Reduction, Stress Management
Volume 43: Body Relaxation
Volume 44: Deep Relaxation
Volume 45: Fear of the Dark
Volume 46: Falling Asleep and Staying Asleep
Volume 47: Compulsive Buying
Volume 48: Restless Legs Syndrome
Volume 49: Bulimia
Volume 50: Anorexia
Volume 51: Overcoming Nightmares
Volume 52: Imagined Deformity
Volume 53: Overcoming Distrust, Finding Trust
Volume 54: Processing Failures
Volume 55: Humiliation, Emotional Hurt
Volume 56: Distressing Compassion, Vicarious Suffering
Volume 57: Self-Forgiveness
Volume 58: Self-Awareness, Self-Confidence
Volume 59: Saying No
Volume 60: Assertiveness
Volume 61: Setting Boundaries and Self-Assertion
Volume 62: Decision-Making Ability

Volume 63: Success Orientation
Volume 64: Ruminating, Circular Thinking
Volume 65: Accepting Pregnancy
Volume 66: Birth Preparation
Volume 67: Spiritual Opening
Volume 68: Joy of Life and Inner Lightness
Volume 69: Patience and Inner Peace
Volume 70: Fibromyalgia and Rheumatism
Volume 71: Irritable Bowel Syndrome, Crohn's Disease
Volume 72: Fear of Nausea, Emetophobia
Volume 73: Stuttering and Cluttering, Speech Flow Disorders
Volume 74: Concentration and Knowledge Anchoring
Volume 75: Vitality and Spontaneity
Volume 76: Searching for Meaning and Finding Goals
Volume 77: Life Crises, Life Events
Volume 78: Workaholism, Goal Obsession
Volume 79: Helper Syndrome, Helpless Helpers
Volume 80: Medication Abuse
Volume 81: Gambling Addiction
Volume 82: Internet Addiction, Smartphone Addiction
Volume 83: Hoarding Disorder, Compulsive Collecting
Volume 84: Conspiracy Thoughts, Overvalued Ideas
Volume 85: Fear of Operations and Treatments
Volume 86: Fear of Aging
Volume 87: Travel Anxiety
Volume 88: Anxiety When Urinating, Paruresis
Volume 89: Fear of Intimacy and Togetherness
Volume 90: Fear of Blushing
Volume 91: Coming Out in Homosexuality
Volume 92: Charisma Training
Volume 93: Migraines and Chronic Headaches
Volume 94: Overcoming Allergies, Bronchial Asthma

Volume 95: Normalizing Blood Pressure
Volume 96: Compulsive Perfectionism
Volume 97: Sports Hypnosis, Motivation
Volume 98: Sports Hypnosis, Performance Enhancement
Volume 99: Determination and Focus
Volume 100: Encountering the Inner Child
Volume 101: Cravings, Binge Eating
Volume 102: Stimulating Metabolism
Volume 103: Bipolar Mood Swings
Volume 104: Borderline, Identity Crises
Volume 105: Hypomania, Euphoria, Mania
Volume 106: Restlessness, Agitation
Volume 107: Nervous Breakdown
Volume 108: Adjustment Disorders
Volume 109: Self-Alienation, Depersonalization
Volume 110: Ending Self-Pity
Volume 111: Primary Gain of Illness
Volume 112: Secondary Gain of Illness
Volume 113: Bullying, Victim Support
Volume 114: Letting Go of Envy and Jealousy
Volume 115: Fear of Spiders, Arachnophobia
Volume 116: Fear of Dogs or Cats
Volume 117: Fear of Strangers, Xenophobia
Volume 118: Excessive Worries, Generalized Anxiety
Volume 119: Strengthening Sense of Responsibility
Volume 120: Unrequited Love, Heartache
Volume 121: Work-Life Balance
Volume 122: Letting Go of Unattainable Goals
Volume 123: Allowing and Accepting Help
Volume 124: Letting Go of Adult Children
Volume 125: Tourette Syndrome
Volume 126: Life Changes and New Starts

Volume 127: Accepting Life in a Wheelchair
Volume 128: Understanding and Overcoming Homesickness
Volume 129: Understanding and Overcoming Wanderlust
Volume 130: Dizziness, Meniere's Disease
Volume 131: Overcoming Aggression
Volume 132: Cutting and Self-Harm
Volume 133: Hair Pulling, Trichotillomania
Volume 134: Postpartum Depression
Volume 135: For Relatives of Dementia Patients
Volume 136: Self-Harm, Artificial Disorders
Volume 137: Activating Self-Healing Powers
Volume 138: Preventing Depression Relapse
Volume 139: Reactive Psychoses, Follow-Up
Volume 140: Obsessive Thoughts and Impulses
Volume 141: Compulsive Checking
Volume 142: Compulsive Counting, Symmetry Obsession
Volume 143: Compulsive Washing, Cleanliness Obsession
Volume 144: Compulsive Questioning
Volume 145: Dissociative Paralysis
Volume 146: Phantom Pain
Volume 147: Overcoming Complaining
Volume 148: Hay Fever, Pollen Allergy
Volume 149: Sexual Abuse, Victim Support
Volume 150: Standing Strong Against Sexism, #metoo
Volume 151: Binge Eating
Volume 152: Overcoming Thoughts of Revenge
Volume 153: Detachment from the Aggressor, Stockholm Syndrome
Volume 154: Courage to Separate
Volume 155: Chronic Fatigue, Exhaustion
Volume 156: Fear of the Future, Existential Anxiety
Volume 157: Excessive Worry About Children
Volume 158: Fear of Failure

Volume 159: Ending Distrust and Control
Volume 160: Dejection, Dysphoria
Volume 161: Boreout, Chronic Boredom
Volume 162: Bipolar Disorders, Relapse Prevention
Volume 163: Mania, Relapse Prevention
Volume 164: Nihilism, Feelings of Worthlessness
Volume 165: Thumb Sucking
Volume 166: Being Brave
Volume 167: Being Proud
Volume 168: Overcoming Shyness
Volume 169: Being Able to Delegate Responsibility
Volume 170: Being Able to Show Emotions
Volume 171: Letting Go of Guilt, Victim Support
Volume 172: Processing Guilt, Offender Support
Volume 173: Mood Swings, Cyclothymia
Volume 174: Lack of Drive, Vital Sadness
Volume 175: Hearing Voices with Reality Reference
Volume 176: Confident Communication
Volume 177: Standing Up for Oneself
Volume 178: Taking New Paths
Volume 179: Confident Job Application
Volume 180: No Longer Being Taken Advantage Of
Volume 181: End of Submissiveness
Volume 182: Depressive Numbness
Volume 183: Mood Drops, Affective Incontinence
Volume 184: Mood Instability
Volume 185: Somatoform Disorders
Volume 186: Stomach Ulcer, Psychosomatic
Volume 187: Accepting Amputation
Volume 188: Overcoming and Letting Go of Hatred
Volume 189: Ending Accusations
Volume 190: Allowing Tears, Being Able to Cry

Volume 191: Finding and Sorting Repressed Feelings
Volume 192: Somatoform Pain
Volume 193: Living Autonomously
Volume 194: Anhedonia, Joylessness
Volume 195: Persistent Sadness
Volume 196: Obesity, Food Addiction
Volume 197: Parents of Abused Children
Volume 198: Letting Go and Letting Be
Volume 199: Childhood Sexual Abuse
Volume 200: Fear of Loss

www.ingramcontent.com/pod-product-compliance
Lightning Source LLC
Chambersburg PA
CBHW030455220526
45464CB00006B/2553